Ketogenic Diet

Your Ultimate Guide for Rapid Weight Loss and Amazing Energy!

Free Bonus

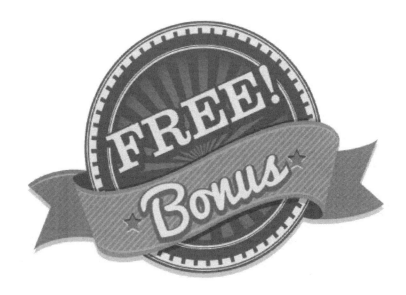

I want to thank you for purchasing this book, hence I would like to give you a free gift in return. Click here or follow the link below to claim your free gift now.
Cheers!

http://eepurl.com/cRXc
Df

The information herein is offered for informational purposes solely, and is universal as so. The presentation of the information is without contract or any type of guarantee assurance.

The trademarks that are used are without any consent, and the publication of the trademark is without permission or backing by the trademark owner. All trademarks and brands within this book are for clarifying purposes only and are the owned by the owners themselves, not affiliated with this document.

Table of Contents

Introduction

I want to thank you and congratulate you for purchasing the book, *"Ketogenic Diet: Ketogenic Diet for Weight Loss and Amazing Energy"*.

This book contains **proven steps and strategies** on how to embark on a dietary journey that is guaranteed to revolutionize your health. In here you will discover actionable and practical information on how to lose fat and improve energy levels. If you have been on other types of diets before and have struggled to shed those pounds or even boost your energy levels, the Ketogenic diet will help you immensely.

So what is a Ketogenic diet? It is simply a diet where a person consumes foods that provide them with more fat, and very few carbs and proteins. In a Ketogenic diet, you get up to **90%** of your calories in form of fats, with the rest being split between the other two macronutrients.

The Ketogenic diet is aimed at causing a shift in the body's utilization away from glucose to fats. In other words, you are causing your body to burn fats rather than what it is normally used to – sugars. During this process, your liver produces substances known as **ketone bodies.**

A Ketogenic diet is very restrictive in terms of how many carbohydrates you are allowed to consume on a daily basis. This level is usually restricted to about **50 to 100 grams of carbs every day.** Carbohydrates have been identified as the cause of most of our society's dietary health issues. This is especially true for processed carbohydrates, which can be addictive and unhealthy. The truth is that most people aren't even aware that all those processed carbs they are eating are making them fat. **All the exercise in the world won't help you lose weight** if you are still consuming large quantities of foods laden with processed carbs. That is why the Ketogenic diet is specifically focused on minimizing the carbohydrate intake.

The quantity of fats and proteins you consume may vary somewhat, but what eventually makes a particular diet Ketogenic is the quantity of carbohydrates it contains. This may seem difficult for some people but it is precisely his measure that makes the Ketogenic diet so effective. Your body simply adapts to the new way of energy production with time. Many people have discovered that the Ketogenic diet is able to help them **burn fat and increase their energy levels** in ways that other diets had failed to achieve.

If you have never heard of or tried the Ketogenic diet, then **this book will unravel it all in a simple and clear manner.** If you already know something about this diet, then this book will still benefit you by going deeper into some of the details that are often left out in other books. You will learn the brief history of the Ketogenic diet, discover what ketone bodies and ketosis really means, and how ketogenesis impacts your body. There are also some **great recipes** that you can sample in chapter 4. In chapter 5 we discuss about the **basic principles of ketogenic diet** and we share some important points about the daily routine and food shopping. Finally, we wrap up with some of the **misconceptions and mistakes** you need to avoid.

I hope you enjoy the book!

Chapter 1: An Overview of the Ketogenic Diet

We all know that a normal diet consist of three macronutrients – carbohydrates, proteins, and fats. The human body generally takes the carbohydrates consumed and breaks it down into glucose, which is the simplest molecule of all. Whenever glucose is detected in the bloodstream, the pancreas automatically produces insulin, a hormone that serves a very important function. Insulin will either transport the glucose to the tissues that require energy at that time, or it may trigger storage of the glucose in form of fat to be used later when required. Glucose is the obvious choice for energy production in the body because it is the simplest and easiest molecule that the body can use when energy is required.

However, a Ketogenic diet advocates for a low carbohydrate intake and elevated fat consumption. One thing to note is that going on a Ketogenic diet and fasting are somewhat similar in terms of metabolic reactions. A Ketogenic diet mimics the metabolic effects of fasting, the main difference being that you will still be consuming food. The goal here is to force your body to produce its energy and meet its calorific demands by burning fats. In order to get to understand just how this entire process works, it is critical that we look at the inner workings of your metabolism.

The moment you stop eating carbohydrates, you will experience a decline in energy reserves. This will happen quickly because your body is used to getting glucose to satisfy its fuel demands. Your body will have no choice but to look for an alternative source of energy. The next best thing would be protein. The only problem with this is that it would lead to muscle wastage, which is something you don't want. Muscles are necessary for all kinds of motion, especially when you consider things from the fight-or-flight perspective.

One viable option is **free fatty acids (FFAs).** Almost all tissues in the body, with the exception of the brain and nervous system, can use free fatty acids. In such a scenario where the body no longer relies on glucose for energy, the brain and nervous system will have to use ketone bodies as an energy source. This is what is known as ketosis. Your body will shift from burning glucose to burning ketones.

Ketone Bodies

What are ketone bodies and where do they come from? Ketone bodies, or ketones, are produced from the partial breakdown of free fatty acids in the liver. When ketone bodies are broken down, the body is able to utilize them as a source of energy. It is important to state that ketosis is a natural process. There are times when you are low on blood sugar or feel as if you are starving, yet your vital organs like the brain still need to function. During such periods of time, ketones are the fallback plan to keep your critical body functions going.

It is also important to note that research has shown ketones to have a stimulating effect on the growth of neural paths within the brain. When your body undergoes ketosis, it is simply following a natural process that helps you burn off the excess fat while improving your cognitive function.

Ketone bodies are not just produced during periods of starvation. There are certain times when the body utilizes both ketones as well as available glucose in order to keep energy levels high. The ketones are used to ensure that there is enough energy for survival. Infants also depend on ketosis as their primary mode of survival. **Mother's breast milk** does not contain much glucose, but rather ketone bodies that are used to provide essential energy. As kids grow up, they are pushed to start consuming a diet that is filled with carbs and sugars. This is when all the unhealthy eating habits start, resulting in weight gain and low energy.

The reality is that a metabolism that burns fat is totally natural and safe. Ketosis has been tried and tested for years and the results speak for themselves. It can be used to treat disorders and is also a good lifestyle to adopt. Once you understand how the Ketogenic diet impacts your body, you will have taken a major step towards your overall health goals.

Ketosis

It is important to clarify the meaning of the term *ketosis* in order to remove any confusion that there may be regarding this term. In most cases, people make the mistake of confusing ketosis and another dangerous metabolic condition that affects diabetics, known as **ketoacidosis.** This condition will be discussed in the next section.

Ketosis can be referred t as a metabolic condition characterized by the burning of fat to generate energy for the body. Instead of breaking down glucose, the body breaks down fatty tissue into ketone bodies. This is what makes the Ketogenic diet one of the most effective ways to use up body fat and thus lose weight. When you start to consume more fats and reduce your carb intake, your body gets used to breaking down fats for energy production.

The moment your body adapts to burning fats that come from foods, it will also find it easier to metabolize the excess fatty deposits around your body. Ketosis as a metabolic process has also been found to repair some of the damage that a carbohydrate-laden diet inflicts on the body, for example, insulin sensitivity and poor metabolic functions. Ketosis is safe and can be used in the treatment of a number of ailments. Compared to taking different kinds of medicines your entire life, ketosis seems like a more sensible solution.

Ketoacidosis

This is a dangerous condition that normally afflicts people who are Type 1 diabetic. A person suffering from Type 1 diabetes suffers from low insulin production. They are also likely to have been consuming a diet filled with carbs for a very long time. Let's say that a healthy individual consumes a meal full of carbs. Naturally, the body will produce insulin to break down the complex carbs into glucose, to be used for energy production.

If a Type 1 diabetic eats the same meal as above, their body will go ahead and break down the carbs to glucose, but there's one problem. They are suffering from inadequate production of insulin. This means that they cannot break down the glucose for energy! The result is that they will eat all they want but they won't have any energy, thus forcing their body to turn to fat as an energy source.

Their body starts to break down fat into ketone bodies for use as n energy source. But therein lies another problem. Insulin is required to regulate the production of ketone bodies, but there simply isn't sufficient insulin to control the process of producing ketones. The result is an overproduction of ketones. Remember that ketones are derived from fatty acids, and from the name itself, you can tell that the body's PH will soon turn acidic. This is what leads to the condition known as ketoacidosis.

Ketoacidosis is characterized by symptoms such as inflammation, dehydration, and swollen brain tissues. This condition can be potentially fatal if not caught and treated in time. For people who are not diabetic, there is nothing to worry about regarding the Ketogenic diet. As long as your body is able to produce enough insulin to control the production of ketone bodies and maintain your health, ketoacidosis is not something to worry about. That is why it is crucial that you consult your doctor before you begin the Ketogenic diet. Even a person suffering from Type 1 diabetes can go on a Ketogenic diet, as there are safe ways to make the diet work for such a patient. For example, if you are taking insulin replacement hormones, you can be able to go on a Ketogenic diet. As always, the most important step is to first confirm with your physician.

History of the Ketogenic Diet
The Ketogenic diet is not a new fad. It has been around for decades, therefore it would be a good idea to review it and

see its progression over the years. There are two ways that the Ketogenic diet has evolved:

1. <u>Treatment of epileptic seizures</u>

The Ketogenic diet has been used in the past to treat children suffering from epilepsy. It has even been documented that fasting was used during the Middle Ages as a way to control seizures. The early 90s saw incidences of children being starved in order to control their seizures, but this was not a sustainable solution.

For this reason, studies were done to look for ways to mimic the effects of starvation while still providing food to the patient. The researchers found out that a diet high in fats, low in carbs, and with minimal protein was the best way to sustain starvation for as long as possible without harming the patient. Dr. Russell Wilder created the Ketogenic diet in 1921. He used it to treat epileptic children who had failed to improve after drug treatments.

The Ketogenic diet disappeared after the 1930s due to the introduction of modern medicines. In 1994, the Ketogenic diet made a comeback thanks to a two-year-old epileptic boy called Charlie Abraham. Neither brain surgery nor drugs could help Charlie, so his father did some research and discovered that the Ketogenic diet had been used successfully in the past to treat his son's condition.

Charlie's seizures were controllable only when he was on the Ketogenic diet. The Ketogenic diet is today widely accepted as a treatment for epilepsy in cases where conventional medicine fails to be effective.

2. Treatment of obesity

For over a hundred years, the Ketogenic diet was used to treat people suffering from excessive weight gain. The morbidly obese patients were normally starved of food, as it was believed that this measure would lead to loss of weight. This form of fasting was reinforced by the fact that ketosis led to appetite suppression and improvement in wellbeing.

The problem with this type of therapy was that the body soon started eating its own protein, mainly muscle tissue. Apart from that, the weight that a person normally loses during fasting is mostly protein and water, not fat. If allowed to continue for too long, it can turn into potential health nightmare!

The 1970s saw numerous studies that revealed the impact of low-carb diets on people with obesity. The conclusion was that, theoretically, consuming a diet containing less than 50 grams of carbs every day would cause you to eat less food. It was around this time that the Dr. Atkins Diet was developed, and it advocated for a high fat, moderate protein, and low carb diet.

It is important to understand how the Ketogenic diet works as well as its history. There is a lot of information that is disseminated out there regarding this diet, so you have to ensure that the information you receive is accurate and credible. This chapter has covered the basics of what you need to know before you get started. In the next chapter, we shall look at the impact the Ketogenic diet has on transforming your body, as well as its many benefits.

Chapter 2: Impacts and Terms of the Ketogenic Diet

Most people have become used to consuming high-carb foods on a daily basis. This means that our bodies become accustomed to breaking down carbohydrates into two components: **glucose and glycogen.** The body does not normally produce a lot of enzymes for breakdown of fats since they are generally stored for future use. Whenever the body detects a reduction in glucose or glycogen levels, it increases the production of fat-burning enzymes.

The Ketogenic diet generally depletes your liver and muscles of their glycogen reserves. The ultimate result will be fatigue, lethargy, dizziness, and even headaches. These are all the effects of a reduction in electrolyte levels. How does this occur?

Carbohydrates are known to cause water retention in the body, especially within the muscles. When you start a Ketogenic diet, you drastically drop your carbohydrate intake, thus reducing the amount of water in the body. This is similar to a diuretic effect. A reduction in water retention in the body causes loss of weight as well as the effects mentioned above.

The solution to this reduction in electrolyte levels is to increase the amount of water and sodium you consume. This is the best way to tackle the initial transition period of your ketosis.

In most cases, people who consume between twenty to forty grams of carbohydrates daily take a minimum of 14 days to experience ketosis. However, there are certain things you can do to essentially quicken the process. Firstly, you can reduce carbohydrate consumption to 15 grams per day. This will ensure that you get into the Ketogenic phase within one week. Another measure you can take is to exercise. Lifting weights and running sprints have been proven to reduce the adaptation time that your body needs to enter ketosis.

The initial days of the diet will be characterized by low energy and strength. However, once your **body adapts** to breaking down fats instead of glycogen and glucose, you will be surprised to discover that you have **more energy than ever before.**

Ketogenic Dieting Principles

In order to get the most out of your Ketogenic diet, you have to understand some of its basic principles and concepts. Most people who want to lose weight tend to focus primarily on bodyweight as the only measure of the effectiveness of a diet regimen. However, this is not a holistic perspective. Another factor has to be taken into account – the ratio of your body fat to your total body weight. This is also referred to as body composition.

Bodyweight versus Body fat

There is a huge difference between losing weight and losing fat. It is surprisingly simple and easy to lose weight within a very short time. If you go for three days without drinking any water, you are likely to lose up to five pounds of bodyweight. This may seem to be a great achievement, but remember, you haven't really lost anything. The moment you start drinking water, you begin to gain back the weight.

What you want to experience is fat loss. This means that you have to make sure that the weight you are losing is from fat reserves and not water or muscle wastage. Another important thing to remember is that as your fat levels reduce, your lean mass should remain constant or increase. However, most people tend to experience some loss of muscle mass as they cut fat from the body. The reason for this is usually a lack of exercise. That is why you are advised to always include exercise in your Ketogenic diet. It will ensure that as you lose weight from fat reduction, your body spares the protein in form of muscle mass.

Body Composition

This is another important factor that you need to keep your mind on. Yes, you may be losing weight, but what about your body fat to bodyweight ratio? Your bodyweight is generally split into two masses – fat and lean muscle. In order to calculate your body composition, you have to find your percentage body fat. This is done as follows:

Body fat % = Fat mass/Total bodyweight

The key thing to remember is that you should always aim to reduce body fat percentage by cutting the fat from your body. Alternatively, you can also reduce your body fat percentage by increasing muscle mass through exercise. The bottom line is that a combined approach consisting of the Ketogenic diet and exercise will give you the best chance of losing fat quickly while boosting your energy levels.

<u>Chapter 3</u>: Benefits of the Ketogenic Diet

The Ketogenic diet is one that should be embraced as a lifestyle. It provides you with many inherent benefits that other high-carb diets cannot. Even if you decide to achieve the state of ketosis for only a brief period of time, the health benefits you will experience will amaze you. Outlined below are some of the benefits that you will enjoy with a Ketogenic diet.

Benefits of the Ketogenic Diet

1. **It elevates your energy production.** Eating too many carbs tends to cause constant spikes and drops in energy levels. The Ketogenic diet eliminates this, thus allowing your body to have constantly high energy and focus levels.

2. **There is a reduction in levels of insulin.** This will allow your body to break down fats more efficiently, compared to a normal high-carb diet. There are also certain hormones that are released when insulin levels are low, for example, muscular growth hormones. Remember, when muscles grow, you lose weight.

3. **A high fat and moderate protein diet keeps you fuller for longer.** You will notice that even when in ketosis, you will not experience the hunger pangs you used to endure when consuming a lot of carbohydrates.

4. **When in ketosis, your body becomes more efficient at generating fuel for its functions.** The problem with a high carb diet is that it makes the metabolic system sluggish and lazy. Ketosis forces the body to up its game!

5. The Ketogenic diet prevents your body from breaking down its own proteins for energy production in favor of ketones derived from fats. This is referred to as **"protein sparing."** This means that muscle tone will be preserved.

6. **When your body is in ketosis, it will trigger the excretion of excess ketone bodies via urination.** We discussed before about ketone bodies being derived from fats, so whenever you remove the surplus ketones from your body, you are actually reducing your body fat percentage. This will ultimately reduce your bodyweight.

Chapter 4: Ketogenic Recipes

This chapter contains some delicious Ketogenic recipes that are also gluten-free. They have been categorized into breakfast, lunch, and dinner meals, as well as some snacks.

Breakfast Recipes

Western Omelet

Servings: 2
Prep Time: 10 minutes
Cook Time: 15 minutes
Nutrition: 72% fat
     25% protein
     3% carbs (5g of carbs per serving)

Ingredients:

- 6 eggs
- 2 tablespoons heavy whipping cream or sour cream
- salt and pepper
- 3½ oz. shredded cheese
- 2 oz. butter
- ½ yellow onion, finely chopped
- ½ green bell pepper, finely chopped
- 4¾ oz. ham, diced

Method:

1. Whisk eggs and cream(or sour cream instead) in a mixing bowl until they become **fluffy.** Add salt and pepper according to the taste.
2. Now add half of the shredded cheese and mix it well.
3. Put the butter in a frying pan and melt it on medium heat. Saute the diced ham, onion and peppers for a **few minutes.** Now add the egg mixture and fry it until the omelet becomes firm. Be mindful of not burning the edges. Take extra care.
4. Lower the heat after sometime. Sprinkle the rest of the cheese on top of the omelet and fold it.
5. Serve it hot. **Enjoy** the delicious and healthy omelet!

Tip!

Try it with a salad, a fresh green one. You can also use some sauce to make it a little spicy if you want to. Personal preference there. **Cheers!**

The Egg Muffins

Serving: 4
Prep Time: 5 minutes
Cook Time: 20 minutes
Nutrition: 72% fat
    26% protein
    2% carbs(2g of carbs per serving)

Ingredients:

- 6 eggs
- 1 – 2 scallions, finely chopped
- 4 – 8 thin slices of air dried chorizo or salami or cooked bacon
- 3½ oz. shredded cheese
- 1 tablespoon red pesto or green pesto (not necessary)
- Pepper and salt

Method:

1. First of all, preheat the oven to 350°F.
2. Chop the meat and the scallions.
3. Whisk the eggs together with pesto and seasoning. Now add the cheese and then stir.
4. Now place the batter in the form of muffins and then add bacon,salami or chorizo.
5. Now depending on the size of the muffin forms, bake them for 15-20 minutes.
6. Serve and **enjoy**.

Tip!

The best part about making these muffins is that **kids just love them**. So, they can be very handy for your kid's lunchbox. That lunchbox will definitely be **empty** after the school.

Salad Sandwiches

Servings: 4
Prep Time: 2 minutes
Cook Time: 0 minutes
Nutrition: 77% fat
    22% protein
    1% carbs(1g of carbs per serving)

Ingredients:

- 3 leaves of cosmopolitan lettuce or romaine hearts
- butter
- Cheese slices
- avocado
- Dried meat
- Tomato

Method:

1. Choose a very **crisp and firm** lettuce variety, preferably cosmopolitan lettuce or romaine.
2. Wash the lettuce thoroughly and use it as a base for the toppings.

Tip!

Play around with the toppings as per your choice but keep in mind the nutrient value also because changing the toppings will also change the nutrient value of the recipe.

Tuna salad and egg salad can be good alternatives. Let the kids select their favorite toppings.

No Bread Breakfast Sandwich

Servings: 2
Prep Time: 5 minutes
Cook Time: 10 minutes
Nutrition: 72% fat
     27% protein
     1% carbs (0g carbs per serving)

Ingredients:

- 4 eggs
- 2 tablespoons butter
- 1 oz. ham
- 2 oz. cheddar cheese or provolone cheese or edam cheese, cut in thick slices
- salt and pepper
- a few drops of Tabasco or Worcestershire sauce

Method:

1. Fry the eggs on **medium heat** over easy. Add salt and pepper according to the taste.
2. Now for each sandwich, use the fried egg as a base. Now place the ham/cold cuts/pastrami on each of the stack. Add cheese now. Now top off with a fried egg.
3. A few drops of Tabasco or Worcestershire sauce will add to the flavor.
4. Serve **hot!**

Tip!

Unsweetened mustard is a very good match with the ham. You can also skip the meat and go with green salad or avocado.

Iced Tea

Servings: 2
Prep Time: 10 minutes
Cook time: 2 hours

Ingredients:

- 2 cups cold water
- 1 tea bag
- 1 cup ice cubes
- Flavorings of your choice, such as sliced lemon or fresh mint

Method:

1. Take half of the cold water in a pitcher and add the tea and flavoring to it and put it in the refrigerator for **2 hours.**
2. Now take out the pitcher and remove the tea bag and flavoring. Replace it with new flavoring if you want.
3. Now add the ice cubes and the rest of the cold water to it and **serve.**

Tip!

You can try this with any kind of tea that you want. You can add lemon or a few leaves of mint to give it a flavor. There are lots of **creative and delicious ways** for it.

Mushroom Omelet

Serving: 1
Prep Time: 5 minutes
Cook Time: 10 minutes
Nutrition: 76% fat
    21% protein
    3% carbs (4g of carbs per serving)

Ingredients:

- 3 eggs
- 7/8 oz. butter, for frying
- 7/8 oz. shredded cheese
- 1/5 yellow onion
- 2 – 3 mushrooms
- Pepper and salt.

Method:

1. Crack the eggs and put them into a mixing bowl. Add a pinch of pepper and salt. Whisk the eggs with a spoon or fork until they become **smooth and frothy.**
2. Add spices and salt according to the taste.
3. Put butter in a frying pan and melt it. Once the butter is melted, pour in the egg mixture.
4. When the omelet begins to cook and get a little firm, but still has a little raw egg on top, sprinkle cheese, mushrooms and onion on top (totally optional).

5. Using a spatula, carefully ease around the edges of the omelet. And then fold it over. When it begins to turn golden brown underneath, remove the pan from the heat and slide the omelet on to a plate.

Tip!

Serve the omelet hot and crispy with some green salad with a **vinaigrette dressing**. So Yummy!

Dairy Free Latte

Servings: 2
Prep Time: 5 minutes
Cook Time: 0 minutes
Nutrition: 85% fat
     25% protein
     0% carbs(0g carbs per serving)

Ingredients:

- 2 eggs
- 2 tablespoons coconut oil
- 12/3 cups boiling water
- 1 pinch vanilla extract
- 1 teaspoon pumpkin pie spice or ground ginger

Method:

1. Take a blender and blend all the ingredients in it.
2. Drink and enjoy.

Tip!

You can replace the spices with one tablespoon of **cocoa or instant coffee**, if you want chocolate or plain latte. **Cheers!**

Keto Porridge

Servings: 1
Prep Time: 5 minutes
Cook Time: 5 minutes
Nutrition: 90% fat
    7% protein
    3% carbs(4g of carbs per serving)

Ingredients:

- 1 tablespoon chia seeds
- 1 tablespoon sesame seeds
- 1 egg
- 5⅓ tablespoons heavy whipping cream
- 1 pinch salt
- 1 oz. butter or coconut oil

Method:

1. Take all the ingredients and mix them in a bowl **except butter.** Let it sit for **2-3** minutes.
2. Take a small pan and melt butter or oil in it on medium heat.
3. Now pour the other ingredients and continue to stir until the porridge becomes firm. Do not let the porridge boil, let it simmer.
4. Serve it hot with melted butter.
5. **Enjoy!**

Coffee With Cream

Serving: 1
Prep Time: 5 minutes
Cook Time: 0 minutes
Nutrition: 93% fat
    4% protein
    3% carbs(2g carbs per serving)

Ingredients:

- ¾ cup coffee, brewed the way you like it
- 4 tablespoons heavy whipping cream

Method:

1. Make your coffee your own way, **the way you like it.**
2. Take a small saucepan and pour the cream into it and heat gently while stirring and until its frothy.
3. Now pour the warm cream in a cup and add coffee to it and stir.
4. Serve it as it is or with a handful of nuts or a little bit of cheese. Enjoy.

Tip!

Add a dark chocolate to your coffee with lots of cocoa solids. This way, when you finish your coffee you will have a **melted treat** for you. Cheers!

Coconut Porridge

Serving: 1
Prep Time: 0 minutes
Cook Time: 10 minutes
Nutrition: 87% fat
     10% protein
     3% carbs(4g of carbs per serving)

Ingredients:

- 1 oz. butter
- 1 egg
- 1 tablespoon coconut flour
- 1 pinch ground psyllium husk powder
- 4 tablespoons coconut cream
- 1 pinch salt

Method:

1. Take a **non stick saucepan** and mix all the ingredients in it over a low heat. **Stir constantly** until you achieve the desired texture.
2. Serve it with coconut milk or cream. A few fresh or frozen berries can be used as a topping.
3. Serve and enjoy.

Tip!

The leftover coconut milk can be reused, put some into your next smoothie. It will add a little fat to it and also thicken it up a bit.

Caprese Omelet

Servings: 2
Prep Time: 10 minutes
Cook Time: 10 minutes
Nutrition: 72% fat
    25% protein
    3% carbs(3g of carbs per serving)

Ingredients:

- 2 tablespoons olive oil
- 6 eggs
- 3½ oz. cherry tomatoes cut in halves or tomatoes cut in slices
- 1 tablespoon fresh basil or dried basil
- ⅓ lb fresh mozzarella cheese
- salt and pepper

Method:

1. Take a mixing bowl, crack the eggs into it and add the salt and pepper according to your taste. Use a fork to whisk until **fully combined.** Add basil to it and then stir.
2. Cut the tomatoes in halves or slice, whatever you like. Dice or slice the cheese.
3. Take a large frying pan and heat oil in it. Now fry the tomatoes for a **few minutes.**

4. Now take the egg batter and pour it on top of the tomatoes. Wait until the batter is slightly firm before adding the mozzarella cheese.
5. Now lower the heat and let the omelet set.
6. Serve immediately and **Enjoy!**

Cheese Omelet

Servings: 2
Prep Time: 4 minutes
Cook Time: 10 minutes
Nutrition: 78% fat
      20% protein
      2% carbs (4g of carbs per serving)

Ingredients:

- 6 eggs
- 3 oz. butter
- 7 oz. shredded cheddar cheese
- salt and pepper to taste

Method:

1. Whisk the eggs until they become **smooth and a little frothy.** Blend in half of the shredded cheddar. Pepper and Salt must be according to the taste.
2. Take the butter and melt it in a hot frying pan.
3. Now pour in the egg mixture and let it set for a few minutes.
4. Lower the heat slightly and continue cooking until the egg mixture is almost cooked through. Now add all the remaining cheese. Fold and serve immediately. **Enjoy!**

Tip!

You can also add chopped vegetables, herbs and even a side of salsa. Use olive oil or coconut oil to cook your omelet for a different flavor.

Raspberry Protein Pancakes

This Ketogenic breakfast dish contains 275 calories in total – 55 grams of fat, 36 grams of proteins, 29 grams of carbohydrates, and 9 grams of fiber.

Ingredients:

- ¼ cup egg whites
- 2 Tbsp Greek yogurt
- 1 scoop protein powder
- ¾ cup frozen raspberries
- 1 Tbsp Cinnamon
- ½ a banana
- 2 Tbsp almond milk
- 1 Tbsp Chia seeds

Method:

1. Grind the Chia seeds.
2. Mash the banana
3. Take a bowl and put in all the ingredients. Leave the raspberries out. Mix thoroughly.
4. After mixing the ingredients well, toss in the raspberries and stir.
5. Sprinkle some Olive oil onto a pan. Pour the mixture into the pan and cook over medium heat until the edges of the pancakes turn brown, then flip.

6. Check to make sure that the middle part of the pancake is well cooked.
7. Serve the meal with the **Greek yogurt.**

The Perfect Bacon and Scrambled Eggs

This delicious Ketogenic breakfast contains 318 calories in total – 26.3 grams of fat, 17.4 grams protein, and 1.8 grams carbohydrates.

Ingredients:

- 3 large eggs
- 1 Tbsp unsalted butter
- Coarse salt
- Ground pepper

Method:

1. Break the eggs into a medium-sized bowl.
2. Take a medium nonstick skillet and place it over low heat. Place the butter in the skillet and allow it to melt.
3. Take a **heatproof spatula** and gently pull the eggs towards the center of the skillet. Cook the eggs for about **2 to 3 minutes.**
4. Add pepper and salt to taste.
5. Serve hot.

Lunch Recipe

Ground Beef Stir Fry

This Ketogenic dish contains 307 calories – 18 grams of fat, 29 grams of protein, and 7 grams of carbohydrates. It serves up to 3 people.

Ingredients:

- 10 ½ oz ground beef
- 2 leaves kale
- 1 Tbsp coconut oil
- ½ cup broccoli
- 5 brown mushrooms
- ½ medium Spanish onions
- 1 Tbsp Cayenne pepper
- ½ medium red peppers
- 1 Tbsp Chinese Five Spices

Method:

1. Chop the red pepper, onions, kales, and broccoli into pieces, and then slice the mushrooms.
2. Pour the coconut oil into a large skillet and cook the onions for **one minute** with medium-high heat.
3. Toss in the chopped vegetables and cook them for another **two minutes.** Keep stirring throughout.

4. Add the spices and ground beef into the skillet. Reduce the heat to medium and cook for about **two minutes.**
5. Place a lid over the skillet and cook for about **10 more minutes,** until the beef becomes brown.

Cocoa Butter Keto Blondies

Servings: 20 blondies
Prep time: 15 minutes
Cook time: 30 minutes
Nutrition: 70% fat
      20% protein
      10% carbs

Ingredients:

- 1/4 cup almond flour
- 2 tablespoon coconut flour
- 1/4 teaspoon baking soda
- 1/4 teaspoon salt
- 6 tablespoon cocoa butter
- 4 tablespoon butter unsalted
- 2 large eggs
- 1/2 cup erythritol
- 1 teaspoon vanilla extract
- 2 tablespoon coconut cream
- 1/2 oz. dark chocolate chopped
- 2 tablespoon walnuts or any nuts or chia (optional)

Method:

1. Firstly preheat the oven to **320°F.** Now line a **baking pan (8*9 inch)** with some parchment paper. Measure out all the ingredients now.
2. Now take a microwave safe bowl and cut the butter and cocoa butter into it. Let them melt in the microwave for

90 seconds. Now take the mixture out and stir the mixture and make sure there are no lumps left. If required, microwave for another **60 seconds** or so. Let it cool now.

3. Take a **hand electric mixer** and mix the eggs, erythritol, and vanilla extract. Now add the coconut cream and mix it again.

4. Now take the cooled butter and pour it into it. Mix it until the mixture gets denser and creamy.

5. Now **sieve and mix** the two flours, baking soda and salt. Add the flour mixture to the cream and combine it well with a rubber spatula.

6. Add the chopped chocolate and stir it well again.

7. Now take the mixture and put it into a baking pan and spread it out evenly, using a **spatula.**

8. Bake it for **30 minutes** in the oven. Make sure that the blondies are a little bit fudgy in the middle. Do not over bake them.

9. When the baking is complete, take out the whole batch from the pan together with the parchment paper and then let it cool. Cut it into **20 pieces** (size and number is your choice) of equal size when its cooled.

10. Serve and **Enjoy!**

Dinner Recipe

Ketogenic Reuben Casserole

This dinner recipe contains 360 calories per serving – 25 grams of fat, 14 grams of protein, 5 grams of carbohydrates, and 2 grams of fiber.

Ingredients:

- 2 cups shredded Swiss cheese
- 8 oz. cream cheese
- ½ pound corned beef
- ½ cup mayonnaise
- 2 Tbsp pickle brine
- 1 can of drained sauerkraut
- ½ cup low-sugar ketchup
- ½ tsp Caraway seeds

Method:

1. Heat the oven to about **662** degrees Fahrenheit.
2. Slice the corned beef into chunks.
3. Put the mayonnaise, ketchup, and cream cheese in a saucepan. Heat the mixture until it melts.
4. Add the beef chunks into the saucepan. Toss in **1 ½ cups** of the Swiss cheese and one can of drained sauerkraut. Stir well.
5. Take the saucepan off the heat and sprinkle the pickle brine.

6. Get a greased dish and pour the mix into it. Add the ½ **cup** of shredded Swiss cheese that was left over. Top it off with the Caraway seeds.
7. Put the dish in the preheated oven for about **20 minutes.** Once the mixture begins to bubble and the cheese melts, remove it from the oven.

Coconut Lime Skirt Steak

Servings: 2
Prep Time: 10 minutes
Cook Time: 40 minutes

Ingredients:

- 1/2 cup coconut oil, melted
- zest of one lime
- 2 tablespoon freshly squeezed lime juice from one lime
- 1 tablespoon minced garlic
- 1 teaspoon grated fresh ginger (I used the fresh stuff in the tube)
- 1 teaspoon red pepper flakes
- 3/4 tsp sea salt
- 2lb grass fed skirt steak (you can cut it into sections)

Method:

1. Combine the coconut oil with lime juice and zest, garlic, ginger, red pepper flakes and salt in a large bowl. **Mix them properly.**
2. Now add the steak toss/rub with marinade.(After you are done, the coconut oil will harden)
3. Now for about almost **20 minutes,** let the meat marinate at room temperature. It is **very important** to marinate the meat.

4. Now take your steak to a large skillet set, which is set over medium high heat. If the steak does not fit then cut it into half. Cut the steak **against the grain.** Some of your marinade can still be stuck to the bowl, spoon it out in to the pan and cook it with the steak.

5. Now cook the steak on each side for about **5 minutes.** Skirt steaks does not take much time to cook.

6. Now slice it and **serve!**

Cauliflower Soup

Servings: 4
Prep Time: 5 minutes
Cook Time: 15 minutes
Nutrition: 90% fat
      7% protein
      3% carbs(5g of carbs per serving)

Ingredients:

- 3¾ cups chicken stock or vegetable stock
- 1 lb cauliflower
- 7¾ oz. cream cheese
- 1 tbsp Dijon mustard
- 4 oz. butter
- Pepper and Salt
- 7 oz. panchetta or bacon, diced
- 1 tbsp butter, for frying
- 1 tsp paprika powder or smoked chili powder
- 3½ oz. pecan nuts

Method:

1. The first step is to trim the cauliflower and cut it into small florets. Cut them small for the soup to be ready faster.
2. Now take a handful of cauliflower(fresh) and chop it into tiny bits.
3. Now sauté the chopped cauliflower and pancetta in the butter until they become crispy.

4. Add the paprika powder and the nuts towards the end and then set aside the mixture and save the fat.

5. Meanwhile, take the cauliflower florets and **boil them** in the stock until they become **soft**. Now add cream cheese, butter and mustard.

6. Mix it with a hand blender. The **more you blend,** the **creamier the soup** will be. Add salt and pepper according to your taste.

7. Serve in bowls, and **top it** with panchetta and cauliflower crumbles in the end.

8. **Enjoy!**

Butter Coffee Rubbed Tri Tip Steak

Servings: 2
Prep Time: 10 minutes
Cook Time: 35 minutes
Nutrition: 75% fat
     21% protein
     4% carbs(4g of carbs per serving)

Ingredients:

- 2 Tri-tip steaks (of course the other cuts of beef would work too)
- 1 teaspoon course ground black pepper
- 1/2 tablespoon sea salt
- 1 package of Coffee Blocks
- 1/2 tablespoon garlic powder
- 2 tablespoon olive oil

Method:

1. Take the meat and let it sit at room temperature for about **15-20 minutes.** Take a mallet and pound the meat to tenderize(optional).
2. Combine all the ingredients in a bowl except steak.
3. Now rub the mixture all over steaks (top, bottom and sides).
4. On a **medium high heat**, heat a skillet with the olive oil.
5. Now add steaks to skillet and cook for **5** minutes on one side. It will also keep the coffee from **burning.**

6. Now flip it and cook on the other side for another **5** minutes.
7. Remove the pan and let it sit there in its own juices. Let it reabsorb them. **Yummy!**
8. Now cut the steak into slices against the grain and then enjoy your **Delicious Piece of Art.**

Tip!

This would also be very delicious with skirt steak also. Cook skirt steak on high because it needs to be cooked shorter and hotter.

Keto Swedish Meatballs

Servings: 4
Prep Time: 20 minutes
Cook Time: 2 hour 20 minutes

Ingredients:

- 2 lbs ground meatloaf blend (or 1 lb ground beef and 1lb ground pork is fine)
- 1 cup shredded mild Cheddar cheese
- 1 large egg
- 1 tbsp water
- 1/4 cup diced onions
- 1/2 tsp ground nutmeg
- 1/4 tsp allspice
- 4 tbsp salted butter
- 1.5 cups chicken broth
- 1.5 cups heavy (whipping) cream
- 1 tbsp Dijon mustard
- 1 tbsp Worcestershire sauce

Method:

1. Preheat the oven to **400°F** and also preheat a slow cooker to low.
2. Now line a big baking pan with parchment paper.
3. Now **combine** ground meat with cheddar cheese, egg, onion, water, allspice and nutmeg in a big bowl.

4. Now roll the mixture into **1.5-2 inch** meatballs and put them on the lined baking pan. Make around **20-25 meatballs.** You might need 2 baking pans depending on the size of your baking pan.
5. Now keep baking for about **20 minutes.**
6. Meanwhile, heat the butter, chicken broth and heavy cream over medium heat in a small skillet.
7. Now it will begin to simmer. Once it starts simmering, reduce the heat to low and let it simmer for about **20 minutes** until it reduces to half. Stir frequently towards the end.
8. Now stir in the Worcestershire sauce and mustard.
9. Now its time to pour the sauce into the slow cooker. Add the meatballs whenever they are ready.
10. Now cook on the low heat for about **2 hours.** It will give the meatballs the time to marinate.
11. Keep stirring after **every half hour,** covering all the meatballs.

Tip!

Do not cook in the slow cooker for more than 2 hours. Cooking more than 2 hours can cause the **sauce to separate.**

*This recipe is not for you if you are a beginner at cooking. This is more sort of an **advanced recipe** and requires a little bit of experience in cooking.

Dessert Recipe

Low Carb Pie Crust

This is a delectable dessert recipe that is used to make miniature tart shells.

Ingredients:

- 2 large eggs
- 4 Tbsp melted butter
- 2 cups almond flour
- 1 tsp salt

Method:

1. Preheat the oven to **662** degrees Fahrenheit.
2. Place the almond flour and melted butter into a bowl and mix them well.
3. Add the eggs and salt as you keep mixing. Ideally, the dough is supposed to pull toward the middle of the bowl and form a ball. If not, add some more flour.
4. Take the ball of dough and put it on parchment paper. Cover it with a sheet of parchment paper.
5. Take a rolling pin and make ¼" thick rectangular shapes. Cut circles in the dough using a biscuit cutter.
6. Line a cupcake pan with cupcake paper and place the dough circles on the pan. Put the pan in the preheated oven and heat until the edges turn golden.
7. **Serve and enjoy!**

Snack Recipe

Kale and Bacon Chips

As a Ketogenic snack, this dish serves up about 62 calories for every cup of kale used. It contains 6 grams of fat, 1 gram of protein, and 1 gram of carbohydrates.

Ingredients:

- 5 cups kale leaves
- 2 Tbsp butter
- ½ cup bacon grease
- 2 tsp salt

Method:

1. Preheat the oven to **662** degrees Fahrenheit.
2. Remove the stems from the kale leaves and chop the leaves into small pieces. Use a salad spinner to wash and dry them.
3. Place the bacon grease and butter in a pan and heat the mixture till it melts. Add the salt and stir.
4. Put all the kale pieces inside a Ziploc bag and pour the bacon grease-butter mixture into the bag. Without sealing the bag, shake the bag until all the leaves have been coated with the mixture. Use your hands to coat the leaves thoroughly.
5. Take a cookie sheet and line it using parchment paper. Place the kales on the sheet.

6. Put the kales in the oven and heat until **brown and crispy.** The smaller bits of kale tend to cook faster so it is advisable to heat the larger and smaller pieces on separate cookie sheets.

Chapter 5: Basic Principles

- **Stick with the basic keto ratio: 61-75%** of calories from the fat, **14-30%** calories from the protein and **6-10%** calories from the net carbs.
- Start slowly. Get the daily net carbs (total carbs without fiber) down to at least less than **50** grams, preferably **20-30** grams. Increase slowly to find the optimal carbs intake for you. Most of the people are able to stay in ketosis at **20-30** grams of net carbs per day.
- Your protein intake should be **moderate**. Try to use your body fat percentage to get the best estimate for your optimal protein intake (**0.6 to 1** grams per pound of lean body mass or **1.3 to 2.2** grams per kg of lean body mass).
- You should try to increase the proportion of the calories that come from healthy fats (saturated, omega 3s, monounsaturated etc.)
- If the net carbs limit is very low (20 grams and below) then try to avoid eating fruit and low-carb treats.
- Eat whenever you are hungry, does not matter if it is a meal a day. Do not let others tell you what you should eat or how often you should eat.
- You do not have to deliberately **limit the quantities** of food that you are consuming, but you should definitely stop eating when ever you feel full, even if the plate is not empty, just save it for later.
- Do not count your calorie intake, just listen to what your body needs and demands. Ketogenic diet and low-carb diets have a natural appetite control effect and you will

automatically eat less. You should keep an eye on your calorie intake only if you reach a weight loss plateau.

- Water is really important in this diet. Increase the intake of water that you have now. You must be drinking 2-3 liters of water everyday.
- Try to eat **real foods** like eggs, meat and non-starchy veggies. This might be contrary to what we have been told for decades but these are very good for you!
- If you want to **snack,** go for healthy foods high in fat (foods containing coconut oil, avocados, macadamia nuts, etc.)
- Try to include some healthy foods like fermented foods, bone broth and offal in your day to day diet.
- Do not be afraid of the **saturated fat** and you can use it for cooking (coconut oil, butter, lard, tallow, ghee, palm oil - organic from sustainable agriculture). No problem in this.
- Always use **unsaturated fats for salads** (olive oil, nut oils, sesame oil, flaxseed oil, avocado oil - organic, extra virgin). Some of them can be used for light cooking.
- Just **avoid** all of the following things:
  - ➤ Processed vegetable oils
  - ➤ Margarine
  - ➤ Hydrogenated oils
  - ➤ Partially hydrogenated oils
  - ➤ Corn oil
  - ➤ Canola oil
  - ➤ Soybean oil
  - ➤ Grapeseed oil
  - ➤ Trans fat

- Try to eat **raw dairy** (none in case of allergies). And look for raw, organic and grass-fed dairy. Just avoid milk (high in carbs) or use small amounts of unpasteurized full-fat milk.

- If you want to eat nuts, try to **soak and dehydrate** them first.
- Never trust the products labeled as "Low Carb". You can not afford to put your health as risk. Labeled products can be dangerous in Ketogenic Diet. Natural foods must always be the priority. Focus on the foods that are naturally low in carbohydrates. Make sure you always opt for real and unprocessed food.
- Labeled products are always deceptive, they are often higher in carbs than they claim. So consuming these kind of products can harm your plans. Labeled products often contain artificial additives which are not allowed in the keto diet. Aspartame (an artificial sweetener) which is present in the diet soda is not at all healthy and has shown many adverse effects on our health. The big companies have financial interests and they deceive the customer in every possible way. So always go for the natural and unprocessed food and do not fall in to the trap of labeled products.

Beware of the hidden carbs and the unhealthy ingredients

- Always read the labels and try to avoid hidden carbs, unnecessary additives, colourings, preservatives or artificial sweeteners. These are found even in chewing gums and mints. They can **trigger cravings** for sugar and they are also not good for health. If you want use sweeteners, go for those with no effect on blood sugar.
- Just avoid everything labeled as **"low-fat"** or **"fat-free",** as it usually has artificial additives and extra carbs. These type of foods also have no sating effect and you will feel hungry soon after you have eaten it.
- Try to avoid the products which are labeled **"low-carb"** or **"great for low-carb diets"**. It has been shown that most of these commercially available products are not healthy. They are also not low carb. They are introduced in the market for financial purposes only. Try to avoid them or choose the best ones only.
- **Medicines:** Cough syrups and drops contain sugar. So try to find sugar-free replacements.

Increase the intake of Electrolyte

We always focus on the **macro-nutrients** (fat, carbs and protein) but neglect the **micro-nutrients** (vitamins and minerals). This is not a good habit. They are equally important and our body constantly requires their intake.

In a low carb diet, there is a deficiency of electrolytes, especially in very low-carb diets such as below 20 g net carbs

Here are a few tips to get your daily electrolytes:

1. **Potassium:** To increase the intake of potassium eat avocados, mushrooms, fatty fishes such as salmon and add potassium chloride to your regular salt (or mix ½ tsp in one litre of water and drink it throughout the day). Be very careful with potassium supplements, do not exceed the recommended daily intake. Never!

2. **Magnesium:** To increase the intake of magnesium one should eat a handful of nuts every day and take magnesium supplement. If you are eating less than 20-25 grams of net carbs daily then it will be very difficult for you to get to your daily targets.

3. **Sodium:** Do not be afraid to use salt and drink bone broth or use it in your everyday cooking.

Always plan your diet in advance and avoid the accidents.

If you want to save your money as well as your time then you will need to plan your diet in advance. And if you are new to this type of diet and lifestyle then it becomes more important for you. Here are some tips before you get started:

- Just get rid of everything that is not allowed on the diet (flour, sugar and sugary snacks, bread, processed foods, etc.) to avoid any kind of temptation. Trust me, if it is in your house, you will likely crave it. This is the only way to avoid the unnecessary **"fridge accidents"**. These accidents may ruin all your efforts.
- Just make sure that some keto friendly food is always available to you like avocado, meat, nuts, cheese, some non starchy veggies or some home made protein bars. Foods that are rich in protein are very sating and they will always help you fight you **hunger cravings.**
- Do you have sugar cravings? Well if you do then I have a **solution** for it. Just drink a glass of water (sparkling or still) with fresh lime or lemon juice and 4-5 drops of stevia. You can also drink some tea or coffee with cream.
- Do not forget to make a list for your weekly shopping. This is very important. Plan your week and then make a

list of things you will require to cook your recipes. Not having the right ingredients when you are planning to cook something is always a pain in the butt so be prepared and plan everything and make a list and then go shopping.

- We all want to save some time and also save some money. For this have hard boiled eggs and cooked meat ready to be used in salad or for a quick snack. Meat (slow cooked) like this one could be used in a lot of different ways (in omelet or on top or lettuce and other veggies). Meats which are suitable for slow cooking are cheaper and they can be cooked in advance. Use slow cooker for this or you can simply cook it in the oven on low-medium covered with a lid.

Chapter 6: Misconceptions and Mistakes to Avoid

If you do your own research, you will discover that there is a lot of **negative information** about the Ketogenic diet being propagated out there. The opposition to this diet is severe, yet the Ketogenic diet is not something new or unhealthy. What is unhealthy and unnatural is the way modern society prepares and eats its foods.

If you plan on going on a Ketogenic diet, you will have to know how to sift out the noise and get to the core of the truth. That is why you have picked up this book. Getting factual information about ketosis will help you avoid some of the many mistakes that people fall into, thinking they are heading in the right direction.

The mistakes people make are usually either dietary mistakes or lifestyle mistakes. You may have been **misinformed about how the diet works,** and even though you are using it, you are not doing so as effectively as possible. It is also possible that though you are committed to the Ketogenic diet, there are some old bad habits that you have refused to let go. Enjoying the full benefits of the Ketogenic diet may require you to change your behavior or lifestyle.

Here are **8 of the most common mistakes** that most people make when on the Ketogenic diet and some of the ways to resolve them:

Inadequate consumption of water, vitamins, and minerals

When in ketosis, never make the mistake of eating insufficient mineral salts, vitamins, or drinking insufficient water. Salt is very important in the Ketogenic diet. Most people tend to view salt as an enemy, but it is still critical to get about two teaspoons of salt every day. Drinking enough water will help you stay hydrated and avoid feelings of fatigue and nausea. Ketosis tends to cause a lot of salts and water to be excreted from the kidneys via urination, so make sure that you are getting enough of your minerals. If you live in an area that is very hot, drink extra water than usual.

Vitamins that you need to load up on include vitamin D. Consume foods such as beef broth or take supplements to boost your salt, potassium, and magnesium intake.

Eating processed Ketogenic food

Do not go to the supermarket and buy a range of processed Keto foods wrapped in packaging. The Ketogenic diet works best when you consume real whole foods. This is the best way to avoid all those hidden sugars and starches that manufacturers tend to sneak into their products. Not only will these cause you to gain weight, they can also negatively impact your general health.

If you can, always try to cook your own meals. If this is not possible, always make sure that you ask whoever cooked the food the ingredients that went into it. If it is a restaurant, check the online menu before you go out. Go for safe foods like salads, broiled or roasted dishes.

If you plan on making the Ketogenic diet a long-term lifestyle, then the best advice is to simply learn how to cook. It may seem time-consuming, but it is well worth it.

Eating too many wrong fats

The Ketogenic diet recommends the consumption of high quantities of fats. However, not all fats are created equal. It is a big mistake to assume that any kind of fat will work for this diet.

Some of the types of fats to avoid include seeds and vegetable oils; especially the ones that come packed in plastic containers. These fats and oils will make you gain weight and damage your health in the long run. Artificial trans fats and partially hydrogenated oils should also be avoided. These are usually found in margarine, cookies, French fries, and many fried foods. The effects of consuming these fats include diabetes, inflammation, and heart disease.

Make sure you always check labels before buying anything. The good kind of fats that you need to be eating can be found in fish, meat, chicken, avocados, walnuts, Olive oil, butter, almonds, Chia seeds, coconut oil, cheese, and many others.

Consuming insufficient amounts of fat

The Ketogenic diet is known to be a high-fat diet, so why would you compromise its effectiveness by not consuming enough dietary fat? This is one mistake that can have the biggest impact on the success of your weight loss goals. The truth is that we have all grown up being told that fat is bad and therefore we should stay away from it. However, you knew from the beginning what the Ketogenic diet was all about. Not eating enough dietary fat is a huge mistake.

People who struggle with weight issues tend to think that fats are the problem, but the truth is that carbs and sugary foods are the real enemy. Take a good look at the kinds of food you eat every meal and you will see a clear imbalance towards excess carbs, especially processed carbohydrates.

Do not be afraid of consuming a lot of **GOOD** dietary fat. In fact, **80%** of your macro nutrient intake should be fats.

Eating too much protein

The Ketogenic diet calls for consumption of moderate amounts of protein. This is because the body cannot make all the amino acids by itself and therefore the diet must compensate for this. Some people tend to consume too much protein than is required for a Ketogenic diet. What is the problem with this kind of scenario?

When you eat a large meal comprising of proteins, more than half of it is turned into glucose. Remember that you are aiming to induce ketosis in your body, so ideally you want your body to break down fat for energy. Eating too much protein hinders this because the body will start to rely on proteins as an energy source rather than fat. You may be surprised to discover that you are on the Ketogenic diet for a long while but aren't experiencing any meaningful weight loss. Furthermore, you will be in a constant cycle of reduced energy levels as your blood sugar rises and drops repeatedly.

It is advisable for you to consume not more than **1.7 g** of protein for every kilogram of your body weight. For a person who is consistently working out, try to increase protein intake to about **2 grams** per kilogram of body weight.

Not getting enough exercise

One misconception that people have against the Ketogenic diet is that you will be so weak and tired from the ketosis that you won't be able to exercise. This is simply not true. A lot of people have discovered that they are actually able to work out even when on this kind of diet.

Let's face it. Exercising comes with **numerous benefits.** You are trying to lose weight by reducing the fatty tissue in your body. You are also trying to generate more energy for yourself. Exercise can help you do both these things and much more.

There are two things you need to keep in mind, however. The first is that the initial weeks of the Ketogenic diet will be very difficult as your body adapts to the new diet system. You will feel weak and somewhat unable to engage in moderate exercise. This is **OK**. Just wait for your body to adapt before you start exercising.

The second thing is that you should adopt some kind of weight training exercises as part of your routine. Cardio and aerobics are great, but lifting weights (keep them light if weight training isn't your thing) will build muscle, and we know that muscle boosts your metabolic rate. A higher metabolic rate will help you cut fat faster.

Skipping your adaptation period

If you are coming from a diet that is high in carbs and now want to switch to a high-fat low-carb diet, you are going to need an adaptation period. Some people make the mistake of jumping right in without gradually easing themselves into the new diet. The result is intense side effects that may make you quit the diet in the initial stages.

It has been noted that skipping the adaptation period may cause intense urges to clear out your bowels. You don't want this to happen when you are stuck in traffic somewhere or are in a meeting. Some people tend to think that there is something wrong with the diet because of this, or that their bodies are rebelling against the diet, but this is not true. The body may be versatile, but it needs time to adapt.

It is recommended that you ease into the Ketogenic diet by slowly lowering your carb intake and increasing your fat consumption over the same period of time. Your body needs to get used to burning fat rather than glucose to produce energy. If you feel hungry during this period, snack on some Ketogenic snacks like nuts, flax crackers, or almond butter. They will help fill you up, and the urge to snack will dissipate once your body finally adapts.

Lack of commitment and goal-setting

If you are going to make the Ketogenic diet work for you, **it is imperative that you stay committed to the cause**. Most people find it hard to maintain a Ketogenic diet successfully because they do not set clear and explicit goals of what they really want to achieve. This is why it becomes harder to stay committed in the long run.

Get a notebook or journal and write down how much weight you plan to lose, how much macro nutrients you will be consuming every day and the time frames for doing so. The success or failure of your goals hinges on how detailed and specific you are.

You also need to get rid of anything from your old carb-filled lifestyle. Clear out your house and give away those foods that do not align with your new **Ketogenic lifestyle.**

<u>Conclusion</u>

Thank you again for **purchasing this book!**

I hope this book was able to help you to appreciate the amazing ways that the Ketogenic diet can help you improve your overall health. You will be able to reduce your body fat levels while getting an incredible boost in everyday energy.

The next step is to take the necessary action and put into practice what you have learnt. Don't forget to consult your doctor before you start any kind of diet, especially if you have some underlying condition. All in all, I hope you enjoyed the book!

Finally, if you enjoyed this book, then I'd like to ask you for a favor, would you be kind enough to leave a review for this book on Amazon? It'd be greatly appreciated!

Click here to leave a review for this book on Amazon!

Thank you and good luck!

45931590R00045

Made in the USA
Middletown, DE
18 July 2017